Binocular Vision Disorder

A Patient's Guide to a Life-Limiting, Often Underdiagnosed, Medical Condition

Binocular Vision Disorder

A Patient's Guide to a Life-Limiting, Often Underdiagnosed, Medical Condition

Denise Drace-Brownell

ELIVA PRESS

CZU 617.7-07-08
D 72

Published by Eliva Press SRL
Address: MD-2060, bd.Cuza-Voda, 1/4, of. 21 Chişinău, Republica Moldova
Email: info@elivapress.com
Website: www.elivapress.com

Descrierea CIP a Camerei Naţionale a Cărţii
Drace-Brownell, Denise.
Binocular Vision Disorder : A Patient's Guide to a Life-Limiting, Often Underdiagnosed, Medical Condition / Denise Drace-Brownell. – Chişinău : Eliva Press, 2021 (Print on demand). – 38 p. : fig.
ISBN 978-9975-909-60-0.
617.7-07-08
D 72

"If you have ever experienced headaches, eyestrain, double vision, blurred vision, general eye fatigue, or a myriad of other common signs and symptoms, you may be one of the many undiagnosed who suffer from binocular vision disorder. Denise Drace-Brownell masterfully dissects binocular vision disorder in this guide to help patients understand what this debilitating condition is, how it is identified, and how it can be treated. As an eye care professional who has diagnosed, treated, and managed this condition in many patients, the research and studies that Drace-Brownell presents in this overview cannot help but make me wonder to what extent eye care professionals may be underdiagnosing and treating this devasting condition. As the demands we place on our visual system continue to intensify in our ever-increasing digital world, it will be critical for patients and eye care professionals to understand and identify this disorder, and treat it effectively through existing or new technologies."

Antonio Chirumbolo, OD
Director of Creative Services
CovalentCreative

"This is a fantastic resource that provides an in-depth look at binocular vision disorder while breaking it down in a way that our patients can understand. It is obvious that we need to create more awareness around this condition, which as Drace-Brownell indicates, is far more common and debilitating than one might think. I believe that literature like this will help drive this awareness, educate our patients and get them talking and thinking about this condition, which in turn will generate a deeper interest in BV disorder within the eyecare community."

Arthur Kim, OD
Founder and Owner
Clearsight Optometry

"One situation that I'll never forget sadly relates to Denise's challenges. I had been tutoring pre-med undergraduate students that were taking college sophomore organic chemistry at the University of Virginia. One student, a very bright young man, came to me privately asking for help, and when I met with him for a lesson review I could see he was visibly upset and held back tears. He had become very frustrated trying to visualize the 3-dimensional structures of molecules, a skill needed to tackle the stereochemistry part of the course. He mentioned he would experience splitting headaches when trying to visualize the spatial arrangements of the atoms from two-dimensional drawings. He also disclosed that he had a vision problem, similar to Denise's. I spent quite a bit of time working with this student using physical molecular models, but after several unsuccessful sessions with me, he decided to drop out of the pre-med program. I felt helpless, and was saddened to see that we'd have one less bright physician joining our society solely because of his vision issue."

Joseph Marasco, Ph.D.
CEO, Verdimine, LLC

"For many years experts told us that our son's persistent reading problem was cognitive. As a family of readers, it was disheartening to see his academic struggles – and how it took away his enjoyment of reading. While he stayed on the Honor Roll, reading assignments were painfully difficult. It was only during his senior year of high school that he was diagnosed with binocular vision disorder. With treatment and home exercises we saw amazing improvements in his reading and writing. Around the same time I became acquainted with Denise Drace-Brownell and her mission to demystify binocular vision disorder, increase awareness, and encourage early diagnosis / treatment. BV disorder affects so many people in the US and around the globe; my hope is that Denise's pioneering work may help other children struggling against eminently treatable BV disorder."

Susan K. Finston.
President, Finston Consulting and Senior Advisor,
Princeton Capital Advisors.

"Denise, you are remarkable."

Dennis Swanson,
Former President of Fox TV Station Operations.

"As is often the case with major breakthroughs, this is a personal story of Denise solving a long standing and almost invisible problem, through her own research that drew upon both her scientific and commercial expertise. Now, having solved her own problem, she wants to share the solution with the world."

John D Graham
Founder, Global Ideation Inc.

Binocular vision disorder is a condition of the eyes, caused by an inability to maintain comfortable sustained focusing at distance or near (accommodation), or comfortable sustained alignment of images which are normally fused to maintain single binocular vision (vergence). The more common symptoms of poor binocular vision include suppression (turning off an image in the brain), double vision (diplopia), blurred vision, eye strain, motion sickness, headaches, fatigue, loss of concentration while reading or working at tasks at near, loss of balance, difficulty seeing in 3-D, poor reading comprehension, and challenges working with abstract formulas used in fields such as science, technology, and finance.

Denise Drace-Brownell
Author

ABSTRACT
BINOCULAR VISION DISORDER

A Patient's Guide to a Life-Limiting, Often Underdiagnosed, Medical Condition

Denise Drace-Brownell identified this unmet need of over 12% of the population in developed countries, with some studies showing a prevalence greater than 30%. These numbers can be expected to increase from society's expanded use of digital devices.

She did breakthrough work in technology with the likes of John Bardeen, the only scientist to win two Nobel Prizes in physics. But because of this underdiagnosed vision problem, her fatigue was so great she had to leave her pioneering work behind.

Decades later she obtained the diagnosis of her condition, invented technology to resolve her challenges, and wrote this patient guide which contains new and valuable information to help patients find their own resolution.

This paper discusses common symptoms of binocular vision disorder, available resources, and typical therapeutic approaches.

Binocular vision disorder impacts corporate productivity, life choices, and ability to make a living. Annual economic damage assessments in the US alone are conservatively estimated at $236.5 billion.

Special considerations concern an individual's limitations in working with formulas, such as those in equations, chemical compositions, spreadsheets, and algorithms. The visual process of reading a formula is different from reading a word. Enhanced visual skills are needed, which are not elaborated upon in this paper. The transformation to a digital age demands a transformation in vision diagnostics, treatments, and technologies.

IMPORTANT NOTE TO READERS

The information in this document is not intended to replace advice, diagnosis, or treatment from a qualified eye care professional. A qualified eye care professional should always be consulted. This material is not intended to be all-inclusive. It contains generally accepted principles and resources to assist patients in finding their own professional assistance.

ACKNOWLEDGEMENTS

Residing in New York City and with associations to MIT gave me access to experts who were critical to the research for this project. Dr. Jeffrey Cooper's insights were of paramount importance. Aside from being one of the world's foremost authorities on binocular vision, Dr. Cooper is a pioneer in developing digital vision therapy systems.

Dr. Aliki Collins' laser-sharp focus and critical analysis made me think beyond my comfort zones and contributed immeasurably to this work.

Nancy Cronin's strategic input regarding technology and intellectual property dynamics concentrated my intellectual and practical outputs. Her husband John's advice years ago kept me working during many a dark hour when some of these findings seemed unbelievable. John said, "If everyone says you are crazy, you are probably on the right track."

Many thanks to Dr. Mark Richard, whose institutional and operations expertise were vital.

The optometric profession's need for additional training in the prescribing and fitting of prism spectacles is a finding I learned from Dr. Antonio Chirumbolo. More training is necessary to fully implement this important therapeutic option. Dr. Chirumbolo provided other valuable practitioner perspectives.

My condition is resolved entirely. It is my fervent hope that this research encourages others to ask for a binocular vision exam to detect this condition, or at the least to bring their symptoms and questions to their eye care professionals, to begin a conversation. If I redirect many of the lives that otherwise would be destroyed through the neglect of this unmet need, then my struggle has been more than worth it.

TABLE OF CONTENTS

WHAT IS BINOCULAR VISION DISORDER?

When we view an object, our eyes must do two tasks. They must fuse the object into one, and they must change focus so that the object is seen clearly. The eyes do this thousands of times a day. In the past, before humans began to actively read and write, the two visual systems that allowed us to complete these tasks were geared to view distant objects, which was ideal for the fisherman and hunter. But with the passage of time, people began to work at varying distances, from miles to inches: first with making tools and weapons, and then extending to reading and writing, and the using of computers and digital devices.

When we view objects at close quarters, as in reading and making tools, our eyes must aim close and point inward. They must converge to focus at close range. The relatively new habits, like reading and using computers, are somewhat different from the older habits at close view, like tool making, in that they are two-dimensional. This adds a new challenge because the two-dimensional items lack the usual cues for aiming and focusing the eyes. Without these cues, the eyes have added strain.

In recent times the strain has been increased even more with the use of formulas, such as those in equations, chemical compositions, spreadsheets, and algorithms. The visual process of reading a formula is different from reading a word. Enhanced visual skills are needed, which are not elaborated upon in this paper.

When fatigue sets in from eye strain, or if there are underlying disorders, the eyes can become misaligned or out of focus. This is known as a binocular vision disorder.

A binocular vision (BV) disorder may involve other issues such as poor tracking and hand-eye coordination, limited depth perception, and limited peripheral vision.

Prevalence of Binocular Vision Disorder

In developed countries at least 12% of the population has some type of binocular vision disorder. Some studies have reported a higher prevalence, such as over 30% of an entire population.[1] With society's expanded use of digital devices, these numbers can be expected to increase.

Symptoms of Binocular Vision Disorder

There are many different types of binocular vision disorders. The most common BV disorders are associated with signs and symptoms, which include eyestrain, double vision, blurred vision, and difficulties with eye coordination and focusing.

Further signs and symptoms include the following:

- Eyestrain or eye fatigue with extended close-up work (reading, computer use)
- Dull headache with extended close-up work
- Double vision (often fluctuating)
- Habit of closing one eye
- Head tilt or head turn
- Car and motion sickness
- Blurred vision (often fluctuating) at near or far distances
- Difficulty switching focus from near to far, or vice versa
- Frequent rubbing of the eyes
- Ability to read for only short periods of time
- Words appear to move when reading

- Losing your place, re-reading, or skipping lines when reading
- Slow reading
- Poor reading comprehension
- Difficulty seeing in 3-D
- Poor eye-hand coordination
- Difficulty processing and recalling information
- Dizziness and loss of balance
- Challenges with navigating small spaces
- Sensitivity to light
- Difficulty understanding formulas such as those in equations, chemical compositions, spreadsheets, and algorithms

People of all ages can be affected by a few or many of these symptoms. The longer and more intense the close work is, the greater the symptoms. These symptoms are more common in patients with a history of brain injury (e.g., head trauma, concussion, stroke, seizures), developmental delays during childhood, autism, and refractive surgery. In addition, binocular vision may worsen with age, leading to an increased risk for falls among older adults. In one study, researchers at the University of Waterloo in Canada found that as many as 27% of adults in their sixties have a binocular vision or eye movement disorder, and 38% of adults over the age of 80 have such a vision disorder.

According to the American Optometric Association, over 60% of children who have difficulty with learning have undiagnosed vision problems which are not detectable by routine vision screenings. The American Optometric Association includes standards for binocular vision testing in their protocols for all comprehensive vision exams. Dr. Carol Scott, a developmental optometrist from Springfield, Missouri, and former president of the College of Optometrists in Vision

Development (COVD), shares: "Considering that 85 percent of all juvenile delinquents nationwide have reading difficulties, it is vital that everyone support the NAACP and ensure that not only are juvenile delinquents and prisoners screened for learning-related vision problems, but all children who have any difficulty with learning, even the bright underachievers."

DIAGNOSING BINOCULAR VISION DISORDER

Initial screening for a BV disorder can be done by an eyecare professional, such as your primary care optometrist or ophthalmologist. More challenging cases should be referred to a specialist. Patients may go directly to a BV specialist if they prefer.

The first step in a BV examination should be a questionnaire which should score or rate symptoms and family history. This is important so that the doctor can quantify the symptoms and compare the findings before and after treatment. Standard BV exams include at least four primary tests: the cover test, measurements of focusing (accommodation), eye muscle teaming, and eye muscle aiming.

A comprehensive eye exam with incorporated BV tests usually includes the following:

Visual acuity: ability to resolve small details

Color vision: screening for any color vision disorder in each eye

Depth perception, or stereopsis: measurement of your brain's ability to see three-dimensional images

Cover test: If an eye is covered and not allowed to fixate or fuse the target, it will move to a position of rest. The further from alignment that the covered eye is, the greater the misalignment of the eyes. By alternating the cover from one eye to the other, the magnitude of the deviation can be determined at distance viewing (20 feet) or near (16 inches).

Near point of convergence: bringing an object slowly towards your nose to assess the eyes' ability to move inwards. The greater the effort or symptoms induced during testing, the greater the relationship between symptoms and testing.

Accommodation testing: using lenses to measure the eyes' ability to focus up close

Vergence testing: using prism lenses to measure the eyes' ability to turn inward or outward together

A Patient Resource for Examinations

The following exam form is an example of the form *required* by the **Department of Defense Medical Examination Review Board.** This form is used by United States service academies, Reserve Officer Training Corps (ROTC) scholarship programs, and the Uniformed Services University of the Health Sciences (USUHS).

Eye Examination Data

	17. Distant Vision		18. Refraction		Manifest	Cyclo	By lens	19. Near Vision		
	Right 20/	CORR to 20/	SPH	CYL		AXIS		20/	CORR to 20/	BY
	Left 20/	CORR to 20/	SPH	CYL		AXIS		20/	CORR to 20/	BY

20. Heterophoria/tropia (Far only)				21. Cover test	22. Color Vision			23. Depth Perception	
ESO	EXO	RH	LH	Pass (Non-Tropia)	Test Used	Results		Test Used	Score
					PIP	No. Passed	No. Failed	VTA-ND/OCT/AFVT	
				Fail (Tropia)	Falant	No. Passed	No. Failed	DPA-V	
					Other (Specify)			TITMUS/STEREO FLY (Arcs per second)	

24. Near Point of Convergence	25. Vivid Red/Green		26. Ocular Motility and Binocularity (Red Lens Test)				
	Pass	Fail	Pass	Fail	If Failed:	Diplopia	Suppression

Some of the important tests included on this form are not always performed in routine eye examinations. Patients can refer this form to their own doctor for initial screening and to inquire about testing.

If you are experiencing symptoms similar to those described in this guide, call your eye doctor to schedule a comprehensive vision exam that includes testing for binocular vision. If you do not have a primary care eye doctor, you can find one here:

Think About Your Eyes: thinkaboutyoureyes.com

American Optometric Association: aoa.org

American Association for Pediatric Ophthalmology and Strabismus: aapos.org

College of Optometrists in Vision Development: covd.org

TYPES OF BINOCULAR VISION DISORDER INCLUDE:

Eye Coordination Problems

One type of binocular vision disorder involves problems with eye coordination. When both eyes are unable to work together, you may notice occasional double vision, words moving on a page when reading, eyestrain, and occasionally the closing of one eye.

If these symptoms most often occur with near tasks (like reading or computer use), you may be experiencing issues with *convergence*, the ability of both eyes to turn inwards together to see single vision up close, or *accommodation*, the eye's ability to adjust focus on objects at varying distances. These disorders include the more common convergence insufficiency and convergence excess, but also include a host of other alignment problems, such as either aiming too close (esophoria); too far (exophoria); or too high (hyperphoria). If the eyes with excess effort cannot be maintained, the eyes may have either an intermittent or constant eye turn called *strabismus*. Again, an eye can turn up or down (hypertropia or hypotropia); outwards (exotropia); or inwards (esotropia). If the turning eye does not suppress, or turn off, the patient with strabismus may see double or blurred vision.

If these symptoms occur off and on with distance or near tasks, and you experience motion sickness, you may be experiencing issues with vertical eye coordination movements due to a vertical eye posture misalignment. In these cases, the blurred or double vision you see may be diagonal or slanted.

Eye Focusing Problems

Another type of BV disorder involves problems with focusing. If your eyes are unable to focus and make images clear at various distances, you may notice symptoms of eyestrain and headaches with near work; the ability to read only for short periods; difficulty switching focus at various distances; or fluctuating blurred vision at various distances.

If, along with these symptoms, you also experience blurred vision up close, you may have an insufficient amount of eye focusing power, also known as *accommodative insufficiency*.

If, along with these symptoms, you also experience blurred vision far away, you may have an over-stimulated or over-working amount of eye focusing power, also known as *accommodative excess*.

Finally, if along with these symptoms you also experience blurred vision at all distances, your eyes may be unable to switch focus to different images, also known as *accommodative infacility*.

Eye Tracking Problems

Yet another type of BV disorder involves problems with eye tracking. If your eyes are unable to accurately track words or moving objects, you will likely notice problems with reading skills, such as frequently losing your place when reading; skipping lines; difficulty copying items from one board or screen onto paper; slower reading speed; excessive head movements; poor reading comprehension; and difficulty reading spreadsheets and abstract formulas.

If these symptoms occur while reading, taking notes, playing sports, or driving, you may be experiencing issues with *saccades,* the ability of both eyes to jump accurately from one object to another, or *pursuits*, the ability of both eyes to smoothly track moving objects.

Amblyopia, or "Lazy Eye"

BV disorder is also associated with *amblyopia*, or "lazy eye." Some children develop amblyopia during early development (birth to age 6) when the brain does not receive equally clear fused images from each eye. If one image is blurred or misaligned, the eyes cannot obtain single binocular vision. The "good" eye actually inhibits the turned and/or blurred eye, and visual acuity is reduced even with correct glasses.

Unfortunately, children who develop amblyopia are often asymptomatic. Occasionally, they may complain of blurry vision in one or both eyes, experience frequent eye rubbing, headaches, or eyestrain. There are no physical signs of amblyopia unless the child has an eye turn which is cosmetically noticeable (large enough for the parents or pediatrician to notice).

As mentioned, amblyopia develops in early infancy or childhood as a result from reduced vision in one or both eyes, due to an uncorrected glasses prescription, strabismus, or a situation where light cannot enter the eye (e.g., cataract, closed eyelid). This results in an imbalance of images between the eyes, causing the brain to ignore the image from the amblyopic eye, also known as *suppression*. Patients with amblyopia typically do not experience blurry or double vision, as they prefer to see only out of the "good" eye.

Uncorrected Glasses Prescription

Nearsightedness, farsightedness, or astigmatism are not considered BV disorders. However, an insufficient or inappropriate glasses prescription, or glasses fitting, can lead to symptoms of blurred vision, squinting, and frequent rubbing of the eyes.

TREATMENT OPTIONS FOR BINOCULAR VISION DISORDER

The most common treatment options for most BV disorders are glasses and contact lenses, vision therapy or orthoptics, and prism glasses. Surgery is considered in some cases, but most BV disorders can be treated with the first set of methods. If strabismus is present, surgery can be an important adjunct to eliminate the eye-turn.

Glasses and Contact Lenses

The first consideration for patients with any BV disorder is to provide you with an accurate eyeglass or contact lens prescription. It is important for both eyes to see as clearly and comfortably as possible before exploring additional treatment options. In some cases, wearing the proper lens prescription alone can alleviate most symptoms.

For patients experiencing eye focusing issues, convergence excess, esophoria, or an esotropia strabismus, an additional near prescription (bifocal or progressive lenses) may help provide clarity and comfort for reading and computer use.

It is imperative to have the correct measurements taken by a qualified optician for your glasses. For instance, failure to take a monocular pupillary distance, which is the distance from the bridge of your nose to your pupil on each side, can make your glasses unwearable. Be sure to select appropriate frames and lenses for your prescription with the help of a trained optician.

For amblyopia ("lazy eye"), it is crucial for the optometrist or ophthalmologist to prescribe the appropriate glasses prescription in addition to any other treatment methods. Studies have shown that wearing glasses full-time alone can improve vision in the amblyopic eye(s) to 20/20, but patients usually need more intensive therapy.

Alternative treatment options for amblyopia include:

- Patching the non-amblyopic eye for a few hours a day
- Using 1% atropine eye drops in the non-amblyopic eye 1–2 days a week
- Adding plus lenses or prism lenses to the glasses prescription
- Enrolling in vision therapy or orthoptics with emphasis on anti-suppression activities
- Surgically removing any object blocking light from entering the eye

Vision Therapy and Orthoptics

A combination of in-office and home-based vision therapy is usually the most effective treatment option for patients with BV disorder.

Vision therapy activities aim to improve visual skills including, but not limited to:

- Breaking suppression (i.e., preventing the "good" eye from taking over) to improve image quality in the amblyopic eye
- Eye focusing skills
- Eye coordination and eye teaming skills
- Depth perception or three-dimensional vision
- Eye movement and eye tracking skills
- Hand-eye coordination skills

The effectiveness and success of vision therapy for each patient depend on several factors, such as the patient's motivation to alleviate symptoms and the patient's compliance with all therapy activities. Also, results are more variable and less predictable in patients with brain injury, so vision therapy is not always an appropriate treatment option for every patient. Note that the primary purpose of therapy is not to build muscle strength but rather to improve the reflexes of focusing (accommodation) and vergence (alignment). This is like learning to ski effortlessly.

Automatic reactions require less effort. Thus, when the therapy is done properly, the effects are lasting.

Prism Spectacles

Prism correction can often help patients experiencing blurred or double vision by decreasing the demand on eye coordination skills. Prism lenses have a thin edge known as the apex, and a thick edge known as the base. When looking through a prism lens, light rays are manipulated so that the image appears to be displaced in a certain direction. The prism lenses are prescribed based on the measured eye misalignment and the prescription results in single vision. A prism effect can also be induced through a variation of the centering of the lens in some circumstances.

Prism spectacles have been prescribed successfully since at least the late 1800s, and modern technology has continued to improve their functionality. One challenge with prism is that patients may adapt to the prism. Thus, initially effective prism may become ineffective, with the patient requiring stronger and stronger prism. That said, prism has a real role in the treatment and elimination of symptoms. Prism reduces the amount of work required to obtain alignment and may be prescribed as a single mode of therapy, or in conjunction with vision therapy and/or surgery to improve the outcome.

Prism can be prescribed as part of your regular glasses as a long-term solution, or as a temporary solution until alternative treatment options become available. Note: prismatic correction is not regularly available in contact lenses, so you would need a separate pair of prism glasses to wear over your contact lenses.

Even more than for non-prismatic glasses, it is imperative to have the correct measurements taken by a qualified optician for your prism glasses. Failure to take a monocular pupillary or pupillary distance can make your glasses unwearable. The appropriate frames and lenses must be selected.

Surgery

Surgery is indicated for eye misalignments that are too large to be properly corrected with glasses or prism lenses or vision therapy. In this case, your optometrist should refer you for strabismus surgery, which is performed by an ophthalmologist. Surgery can be an important part of the treatment plan because it can eliminate or reduce the size of an eye turn permanently.

FURTHER RESOURCES

In addition to the symptoms discussed here, patients with brain injury, developmental delays during childhood, and autism may likely experience other cognitive and visual perceptual difficulties. The following organizations are good resources for additional information about BV disorder:

American Optometric Association

The American Optometric Association (aoa.org), founded in 1898, is a leading authority on vision care, representing more than 44,000 doctors of optometry (OD), optometric professionals, and optometry students.

Their website lists optometrists practicing within your community.

The College of Optometrists in Vision Development (COVD)

The College of Optometrists in Vision Development (covd.org) is a non-profit, international association of eye care professionals offering services that specialize in behavioral and developmental vision care, vision therapy, and neuro-optometric rehabilitation.

Their directory connects you with optometrists providing vision therapy services within your community.

The American Association for Pediatric Ophthalmology and Strabismus (AAPOS)

The mission of the American Association for Pediatric Ophthalmology and Strabismus (aapos.org) is to promote the highest quality medical and surgical eye care worldwide for children and for adults with strabismus.

Their website includes a directory to find a pediatric or adult strabismus medical doctor in your community.

The American Academy of Ophthalmology

The American Academy of Ophthalmology (aao.org) is the world's largest association of eye physicians and surgeons, and provides patient education on the importance of eye health.

On their website, you can find patient information on eye health and a directory to find an ophthalmologist within your community.

The Optometry Extension Program Foundation (OEPF)

This international organization provides advanced education on vision, the visual process, and clinical care to optometrists.

Optometrists associated with the OEPF often have additional experience and knowledge in vision therapy services for children with behavioral or learning disabilities, autism, and developmental delays.

The website (oepf.org) does not offer educational resources for the general public, but it does offer a directory to find an optometrist in your community.

InfantSEE®

InfantSEE® (infantsee.org) is a public health program designed to ensure that eye and vision care becomes an integral part of infant wellness care.

Under this program, optometrists provide no-cost comprehensive eye and vision assessments for infants 6–12 months old, regardless of a family's income or access to insurance coverage.

Their website includes a directory to find an InfantSEE® provider in your community.

Vision Therapy Canada

Vision Therapy Canada (visiontherapycanada.com) is a Canadian association dedicated to enhancing education and awareness of vision therapy and rehabilitation in optometry.

Their website includes a directory to find an optometrist offering vision therapy services in your community.

The British Association of Behavioural Optometrists

The British Association of Behavioural Optometrists (babo.co.uk) is a network of British optometrists with special interests in vision and vision-related learning disorders.

They provide patient information on vision problems and offer a directory to find an optometrist providing vision therapy services in your community.

They also offer a checklist of symptoms related to vision disorders for you to bring to an optometrist.

GLOSSARY OF TERMS

Accommodation: The eye's ability to adjust focus on objects at varying distances. See *near point of accommodation* and *accommodative facility*.

Accommodative facility: The eye's ability to repeatedly change focus from one distance to another.

Amblyopia: A condition, commonly known as **lazy eye**, in which vision is reduced in one or both eyes as a result of interference with normal visual development during the early years. The most common causes of amblyopia are strabismus (eye turn) or anisometropia (different eyeglass prescription in each eye). It is estimated that three percent of children under age six have some form of amblyopia.

Anisometropia: A condition in which each eye has a different *refractive error* (prescription), such as mild and extreme nearsightedness, or even nearsightedness in one eye and farsightedness in the other.

Asthenopia: A condition, also called eye strain, that manifests through non-specific symptoms such as fatigue, pain in or around the eyes, blurred vision, headache, and occasional double vision. BV disorder often results in asthenopia.

Astigmatism: A condition caused by an irregular curvature of the eye's cornea or lens. With astigmatism, you have blurred or distorted vision at near and far distances. Astigmatism is very common.

Behavioral optometry: An international branch of optometry that specializes in the practice of vision therapy. Behavioral optometrists (also called developmental optometrists) will sometimes consider how environmental, nutritional, and/or behavioral factors affect visual health.

Binocular depth perception: The ability to visually perceive three-dimensional space and the ability to visually judge relative distances between objects. A result of successful stereo vision, it is a visual skill that aids accurate movement in three-dimensional space.

Binocular vision: Vision that results from both eyes working as a team, where both eyes work together smoothly, accurately, equally, and simultaneously.

Convergence: The ability of both eyes to turn inward together, which enables both eyes to be looking at the exact same point in space. This skill is essential to reading. Not only is convergence essential to maintaining attention and single vision for short periods, but it is also vital to the ability to maintain convergence comfortably for long periods of time while engaged in reading or other tasks.

Divergence: The ability of the eyes to turn outward together to enable them to both look farther away. The opposite of *convergence* (see above). The sustained ability to make rapid convergence and divergence movements is essential for efficient learning and general visual performance.

ECPs: Eye Care Professionals. Encompasses *ophthalmologists, optometrists, opticians,* and others who work in the eyecare industry.

Esophoria: A tendency of the eyes to deviate inward.

Exophoria: A tendency of the eyes to deviate outward.

Eye movement skills: A term covering the whole range of eye movement skills required for efficient vision. These skills include *pursuit eye movements, saccadic eye movements, fixation skills,* and *ocular motilities.*

Fixation skills: The ability to look at an object long enough to enable recognition or cognition. Poor fixation skills often lead to poor attention and performance, especially at near-related tasks.

Near point of accommodation: The closest distance from the eyes that reading material can be read. This distance varies with age. It is often measured in each eye separately and then both eyes together. The results are compared to one another. See *accommodation* and *accommodative facility*.

Ocular motilities: A term used to describe the range of eye movements. These movements are controlled by six muscles of each eye known as extraocular muscles. Defects in any one of the muscles can cause inefficiencies in eye movement control and increased effort to maintain comfortable, clear, single vision.

Oculomotor skills: The ability to track or follow a moving object and the ability to move the eyes accurately and smoothly from one point to another. These skills are vital in activities like reading.

Ophthalmologist: An *ECP* who is a trained medical or osteopathic doctor specializing in diseases of the eye and eye surgery. An ophthalmologist may also prescribe and fit eyeglasses and contact lenses to correct vision problems.

Optician: An *ECP* who understands how to read a prescription for glasses and who fits and dispenses spectacles according to the prescription.

Optometrist: An *ECP* qualified to diagnose visual health problems, prescribe spectacles and contact lenses, and dispense low vision aids. Some practitioners also offer *vision therapy*.

Orthoptics: Medical term for vision therapy intended to improve fusion and eliminate suppression.

Peripheral vision: The ability to see, or be aware of, what exists around us or to the sides of us. Defects in this ability can be caused by a variety of eye diseases, or something as simple as poor eyeglasses. Good peripheral vision is essential for driving, sports, reading, and general situational awareness. Peripheral vision can be tested using visual field-testing instruments.

Presbyopia: The loss of the eye's ability to change its focus to see near objects and part of the natural aging process of the eye. It is not a disease and can be easily corrected with glasses. Presbyopia generally starts to appear around age 40.

Prism eyeglasses: Eyeglasses that incorporate a wedge-shaped optical component known as a prism. Like a triangle, the thinnest edge of the prism is referred to as the apex, and the thickest edge is referred to as the base. When a ray of light passes through a prism, the ray is deviated toward the base of the prism. When looking through the prism, however, the image appears to be displaced toward the apex because the image appears to originate from the direction of the deviated light ray. The orientation of a prism effect relative to the line of sight of the wearer is specified by the direction of the base of the prism. A prescription for prism correction can be up or down, in or out, or a combination. The prism correction brings the line of sight between the two eyes in common, lessens the misalignment, and often eliminates it. A prism effect can also be induced through a variation of the centering of the lens in some circumstances.

Pupillary distance (PD): The distance in millimeters between the center of one pupil to the center of the other. Having a correct PD measurement on your glasses prescription ensures that you are looking through the ideal spot in your lenses. A PD measurement should also include a **mono-pupillary measurement**, which is the distance from the bridge of your nose to your pupil for each eye. A monocular PD measurement will be two numbers.

Pursuit eye movements: The ability to move the eye to remain in accurate visual contact with a moving object within the visual field. This includes the ability to perform this task not only when the head and body are stationary, but also when the head and body are moving.

Refraction: The part of an eye examination that determines the *refractive error*.

Refractive error: The measure of the error of focus of an eye compared to an assumed normal point of zero. The error is measured in diopters. The refractive error will include measurements for myopia (near sight), hypermetropia (distance sight), astigmatism, and presbyopia (the loss of focusing power, due to age, for near work).

Saccadic eye movements: Eye movements where the eyes jump quickly from one object to another, such as moving fast to look directly at an object approaching from one side, as when one is driving or reading. Saccadic eye movements are usually fast and sequential in nature. Problems may arise when the saccadic movement is consistently over- or under-shooting, which can cause loss of comprehension and fluency in reading, or a constant feeling of losing one's place.

Snellen chart: A Snellen chart is a standardized eye chart used to measure visual acuity or clarity of vision. The chart measures vision acuity at a distance of 20 feet (6 meters), hence the term "20/20" vision. The chart tests whether a patient sees at 20 feet what is considered to be standard in the population. Snellen charts do *not* measure binocular vision. An over-reliance on Snellen charts is often cited as an important reason for the under-reporting of BV disorder.

Spatial skills: The ability to relate to and to judge distances of surrounding areas and objects. Spatial skill affects practical skills like handwriting, body posture, and balance.

Stereo vision (stereopsis, or stereoscopic vision): Relative depth produced by the slightly different images produced by the lateral separation of our eyes.

Strabismus: A visual defect in which one of the eyes points in different directions. One eye or both may turn in (esotropia), out (exotropia), up or down (hypertropia), or a combination of these. Because of this condition, both eyes do not always aim simultaneously at the same object. Also called "crossed eyes" or "wandering eye," these eye misalignments are not always obvious to the casual observer. However, the mis-aiming results in diminished stereo vision and binocular vision if the eye turn is constant.

Vertical heterophoria: A vertical misalignment of the eyes.

Vision therapy (also known as vision training): A type of vision training involving exercises aimed at improving visual skills, such as eye-teaming, binocular coordination and depth perception, focusing, and "hand-eye" or "vision-body" coordination.

ENDNOTES

Footnotes and Additional Commentary

Please note: The following is only representative of the significant data available.

1.　*The Optometrists' Network* is a network of interconnected patient education and optometric websites which educate the public about visual health and the unique aspects of optometric care. Their public health mission is supported by its members who are licensed doctors of optometry. Founded in 1996, the Optometrists' Network now uses the statistic that at least 12% of the population has some type of problem with binocular vision.

The Eyecare Trust in the UK also uses the 12% prevalence statistic: "However, more than one in ten of us (12%) has a visual impairment that means our brains are unable to correctly process the individual images that are transmitted to it via our left and right eyes. This leads to an inconsistency in viewing the three spatial dimensions (height, width, and depth) required to enjoy 3-D films in all their glory. You may not have realized that you have poor binocular vision before, because your brain will often try to compensate for any visual inadequacies."

A study by Dr. Dominick Maino suggests that up to 56% of the population between 18 and 38 could have an issue with binocular vision disorder. As Dr. Maino points out, even if these numbers are off by 50%, they are still large numbers (Maino, D. The Binocular Vision Dysfunction Pandemic. Optom Vis Dev 2010; 41(1):6-13). Other studies show similar troubling statistics. For example, Hokoda (1985) found that 21% of a normal population demonstrated both symptoms and clinical findings of BV disorder (J Am Optom Assoc 1985; 56:560-2). Sixty-five students were selected from a group of second-year university students with no uncorrected refractive errors, healthy eyes, and no strabismus or amblyopia. Some 32.3% of the subjects showed general binocular dysfunction (Porcar, *et al.* Prevalence of general binocular dysfunctions in a population of university students. Optom Vis Sci 1997; 74 (2):111-3).

In lower socioeconomic populations the prevalence is higher. Dr. Antonia Orfield conducted a study of children in an urban vision clinic. Dr. Orfield tested over 800 children and found that over 50% of the children failed the comprehensive vision exam. Most of these students who failed had 20/20 eyesight, an evaluation that merely checks for seeing letters at a distance but does not pick up visual problems or lack of fusion at a close range, which is the range required for reading (J Optom Vis Dev 2001; 32:114-41).

BV disorder is exacerbated by middle-aged vision challenges, especially presbyopia. Binocular vision worsens with age. The results of a study from researchers at Canada's University of Waterloo found that as many as 27% of adults in their seventies have a binocular vision or eye movement disorder, and 38% of adults over 80 have such a vision disorder.

In the studies cited, most cases of BV disorder had been unknown to the patients. Similar data have been collected for the strabismus and amblyopia populations. Strabismus is conservatively estimated to be at least 3% of population, but less than 1% is identified. Repka and colleagues found that only .68 of 1% of Medicare beneficiaries (age 65 and older) in 2010 were diagnosed with strabismus (Repka MX, *et al.* Strabismus among aged fee-for-service Medicare beneficiaries. J AAPOS 2012; 16: 495-500).

Amblyopia has a 3% prevalence in the population. Incidence would be reduced by 50% with proper diagnosis and treatment (William E. Gibson, "Economic Analysis of the Consequences of Failure to Prevent Childhood

Blindness from Amblyopia," a study and publication of the Children's Eye Foundation, 2011). Note: The Children's Eye Foundation (CEF) is the foundation of the American Association for Pediatric Ophthalmology and Strabismus (AAPOS). With approximately 1,200 members representing 41 countries, AAPOS is the world's largest physician organization dedicated to children's eye care and adults with strabismus.

Publisher: Eliva Press SRL

Email: info@elivapress.com

www.ingramcontent.com/pod-product-compliance
Lightning Source LLC
Chambersburg PA
CBHW072141150726
48002CB00004B/1575